D1479272

DIVINE ENCOUNTERS *on a* CANCER FLOOR

Real-life Stories from an Oncology Nurse

TAMMY MOSER

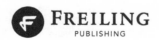

FREILING
PUBLISHING

Copyright © 2022 by Tammy Moser
First Paperback Edition
All rights reserved. No part of this publication may be reproduced,

distributed, or transmitted in any form or by any means, including
photocopying, recording, or other electronic or mechanical methods,
without the prior written permission of the publisher, except in the
case of brief quotations embodied in critical reviews and certain other
noncommercial uses permitted by copyright law.

For permission requests, write to the publisher, addressed
"Attention: Permissions Coordinator," at the address below.
Some names, businesses, places, events, locales, incidents,
and identifying details inside this book have been changed
to protect the privacy of individuals.

Bible versions used:

The Amplified Bible, Classic Edition (AMPC). Copyright © 1954, 1958,
1962, 1964, 1965, 1987 by The Lockman Foundation.

The Holy Bible, New Living Translation (NLT).
Copyright © 1996, 2004, 2015 by Tyndale House Foundation.
Used by permission of Tyndale House Publishers, Inc.,
Carol Stream, Illinois 60188. All rights reserved.

The Holy Bible, New International Version®, NIV® Copyright © 1973, 1978,
1984, 2011 by Biblica, Inc.® Used by permission.
All rights reserved worldwide.

The Holy Bible, English Standard Version. ESV® Text Edition: 2016.
Copyright © 2001 by Crossway Bibles, a publishing ministry of
Good News Publishers.

New English Translation (NET) NET Bible®. Copyright ©1996-2017 by
Biblical Studies Press, L.L.C. http://netbible.com All rights reserved.

New American Standard Bible® (NASB), Copyright © 1960, 1971, 1977,
1995, 2020 by The Lockman Foundation. All rights reserved.

The New King James Version® (NKJV). Copyright © 1982
by Thomas Nelson. Used by permission. All rights reserved.

Revised Standard Version of the Bible (RSV). Copyright © 1946, 1952, and
1971 the Division of Christian Education of the National Council of the
Churches of Christ in the United States of America. Used by permission.
All rights reserved.

Published by Freiling Publishing,
a division of Freiling Agency, LLC.

P.O. Box 1264
Warrenton, VA 20188

www.FreilingPublishing.com

PB ISBN: 978-1-956267-87-7
eBook ISBN: 978-1-956267-88-4

Printed in the United States of America

Dedication

I WILL ALWAYS be grateful for my patients, their families, and dedicated colleagues, past and present. You have contributed to the beauty of my life's story and destiny. And, most importantly, I'm grateful for my Lord and Savior, Jesus Christ, who has guided, strengthened, and carried me through many days when I didn't think I could take another step or write another word. You alone are worthy of all my praise!

SOLI DEO GLORIA

Have You Ever Encountered an Angel?

ONE DAY, WHILE standing outside the metro in Washington, D.C., I spoke to a gentleman who I believe was an angel, but I am not entirely sure. However, a patient of mine once said, "I saw your guardian angel, and her name was **FAITH**."

> Are not the angels all ministering spirits (servants) sent out in the service [of God for the assistance] of those who are to inherit salvation? (Hebrews 1:14 AMPC)

Contents

Acknowledgments

I AM DEEPLY grateful for the coaching and encouragement of Dr. Temitope Keku. You inspired me to capture the vision, get started, and believe in myself. And for Dr. Pao-Hwa Lin, whose weekly probing question, "How is the book going?" helped me to keep working and have the courage not to give up. Also, to my dear friends Bernice, Cheryl, and Lois, whose reading and editing advice helped pave the way to a finished manuscript. I am deeply thankful for each of you and all of your prayers!

Mom, Dad, Eddie, Kelli, Taylor, Luke, Whitney and Avery.

Love you all!
Aunt Tam

Introduction

HAS YOUR LIFE ever taken an unwanted or unexpected turn? Most of us have experienced times like this if we have lived long enough. As a new nurse working in an Oncology Unit, I walked through the corridors and rooms of many people going through times of unchartered waters. They were facing deadly diagnoses but came to us with hearts full of hope for a cure while taking experimental therapy.

I was also walking down a path I had never dreamed of and was stepping out in faith to follow what I believed God was calling me to do. It involved moving to a big city, having roommates I barely knew (I am happy to say we are still friends), and taking on responsibilities I had never encountered in my working career. It was exciting, scary, and quite often felt uncertain. Sometimes, I would have dreams of forgetting to check in on a patient throughout my shift, sending me into a state of sheer panic. It felt more like a nightmare than a dream when I woke up. I thought I would be in my internship for only nine months and return home, but I stayed for nine and a half years working at a hospital in Bethesda, Maryland, near our nation's capital.

Looking back over those years, I realized these stories needed to be written and shared. I couldn't allow the memories of these precious people to be forgotten. Their tremendous courage, strength, and faith carried them through their unexpected events in life. I experienced the incredible privilege of walking closely by their side in perhaps one of the most vulnerable times in their lives. Their trials and suffering made their faith even stronger for many of them. These are the stories I want to share with you.

Before we get started, I wonder if you have ever seen the painting or a photo of Michelangelo's *The Creation of Adam*, which forms part of the Sistine Chapel's ceiling. Adam is reclining on the earth, completely relaxed with his arm resting on his knee and his hand draped downward. God is moving toward Adam intentionally, his outstretched arm and finger reaching, pointing to try and touch him. I love this painting because it reveals God's and man's nature. God is always reaching out to us; he came as a baby, grew up as a man, and sent his Holy Spirit to inhabit his believers while we live on this earth. He created us, this world, and desires to be near us now and always. I witnessed this daily with my patients as they lived out their faith amid suffering.

I pray that you will encounter him reaching down to you through these stories but, unlike Adam in the painting, may you reach back and discover that he wants to hold you in his arms!

> He tends his flock like a shepherd: he gathers the lambs in his arms and carries them close to his heart; he gently leads those that have young. (Isaiah 40:11 NIV)

Kicked Out of the Nest

Seek his will in all you do, and he will show you
which path to take. (Proverbs 3:6 NLT)

IT WAS MY first day off orientation. I was on my own
as a new nurse, working in a surgical oncology unit on
the second floor of a hospital in Maryland. I always had
backup resources, but now it was time for me to learn
to fly by myself, just like a young bird shoved out of her
nest. I was scared, but I imagine all new nurses experience this feeling to some degree. My preceptor, however,
was confident that I was ready, or she would never have
approved of my independence.

My first assignment was Mr. Garner, an elderly
gentleman from Kentucky with metastatic renal cell
cancer. He came to us with hope for a cure, that his
cancerous tumors would shrink, and that he would have
more time to live with the wife he dearly cherished.

If I close my eyes today, I can still see his face and
hear the sound of his voice. He was such a gentle soul
and trusted me completely with his care, even more than
I trusted myself at this early stage in my career. But I

didn't dare share this with him. His wife was always by his side and lovingly called me his other girlfriend since we spent so much time together. We all connected so well, having our southern heritage in common.

Mr. Garner settled into his room, and after being examined by his physician, I checked his vital signs and started his IV. He was then ready to begin his Interleukin therapy. Every eight hours, he would get a new dose of IL2 if his body could tolerate the side effects without causing severe harm. Of course, we gave him a great deal of education regarding the potential adverse reactions; still, I don't imagine he could anticipate how sick he would possibly feel from these treatments.

Almost immediately after administration of immunotherapy in a patient, flu-like symptoms would begin to manifest. We gave multiple medications to help eliminate and minimize these symptoms, and we monitored every patient very carefully during the ongoing therapy. We tracked the patient's heart rate, temperature, and blood pressure every four hours. As new symptoms occurred, we would administer additional medications to help ease the severity of the patient's reactions. It was rigorous nursing care, rarely allowing a moment to sit down during the shift, as is the case for most nurses these days.

In spite of his cancer and intensive treatment, Mr. Garner never complained about anything. Not ever. He was a remarkable man and was grateful for everything we did for him. I remember praying for his healing day after day as I administered his therapy. He responded extremely well to his first round of immunotherapy and returned for continued treatments over many months. Eventually, I would learn that my first patient had a complete response to our experimental treatments.

I had met Mr. Garner back in 1992, and after that, I received cards from his wife from time to time to give me an update about his health and how they were doing. In December of 2000, I got a Christmas card from her saying, "Tom went back to NIH for our clinic visit in September and, as always, got a good report. After this visit, Dr. Rosenberg released him and told him to get his x-rays every two to three years in Kentucky. NIH has been a miracle for us, and you were part of that miracle." I don't take credit for anything and honestly believe the Lord chose to place me there, orchestrate my steps, and allowed me to pray for this humble, gentle soul who needed medical treatment and prayers.

The Bible commands us, "And pray in the Spirit on all occasions with all kinds of prayers and requests. With this in mind, be alert and always keep on praying for all the Lord's people" (Ephesians 6:18 NIV). It is comforting to realize that I had a small part to play in this gentleman's life to help bring about the Lord's will. I just did what I thought the Lord was asking me to do, and God did the rest.

Of course, many players were on this team: scientific researchers behind the scenes working day and night, attending surgeons, residents in training, other nurses on our unit, social workers, dieticians, phlebotomists, environmental services, unit secretaries, and volunteers. We were a village, and it certainly took every one of us to make it all come together to benefit our patients.

What about you? I am confident that you also are given chances every day in your life to make a difference for someone else. Will you embrace these opportunities as they come your way, even if they go unnoticed or unappreciated? The Lord promises, "And if anyone gives even a cup of cold water to one of these little ones who is my disciple, truly I tell you, that person will certainly not lose their reward" (Matthew 10:42 NIV). Even if no other human being notices our serving, we can be comforted that the Lord, indeed, sees all that we do.

Angels among Us

So do not fear, for I am with you; do not be dismayed, for I am your God. I will strengthen you and help you; I will uphold you with my righteous right hand. (Isaiah 41:10 NIV)

CANCER DOES NOT have biases and shows no favorites. Sadly, it strikes at every age in the lifespan of the human race and has no respect for persons, culture, or income level. All the money and resources in the world cannot stop someone from getting this disease.

I made rounds in the early hours of the morning after getting a report from the night shift nurses on each of my patients. As I popped into one particular room, I quickly introduced myself to a young woman in her twenties who was lying in bed anxiously waiting for her therapy to start. With the appearance of a gentle giant compared to her tiny frame, her husband sat quietly beside her. He barely spoke a word, but he didn't need to because his presence was comforting enough, even for me, though I just met them.

Shelly had a rare type of cancer that affected her connective tissue, and she needed a particular chemotherapy drug called Adriamycin. It is still in use today and is considered a vesicant, which can cause extensive tissue damage and blistering to skin and muscle if it leaks out of the vein when being administered. I had seen photos of patients' arms where this leakage had occurred, and the drug had caused severe damage down to the bone. All doctors and nurses must be specially certified to administer this medication.

I explained to Shelly all the details of what I would do before getting started. I had completed my training but had never given this type of chemotherapy alone, so my preceptor was observing and instructing me. While interacting with Shelly, I realized she was a Christian, so I asked if she would like to pray before we started. She agreed, and as I began, big tears rolled down her cheeks. I sensed she was afraid and probably overwhelmed. She didn't verbalize anything, but I could only imagine what thoughts and feelings were running through her mind. After inserting the butterfly needle into her small vein, I carefully and slowly started administering the medicine.

The Lord gave me the grace to be a reassuring and calming presence during the entire treatment. Honestly, as much as she was afraid to receive this drug, I was scared to give it, knowing the devastating consequences that could happen if not administered correctly. God's grace is sufficient, no matter the test or trial we are going through or which side of the fence we are sitting on.

I continued to give Shelly her treatments over the weeks and months to come. Thankfully, I successfully administered them without any serious consequences. I am confident the Lord had his angels watching over both of us, and she later relayed this same message to me in a card she sent. I haven't been in touch with Shelly, but with the help of the internet, I found her photograph and a small story about her cancer history. She is well and living a full life more than twenty years after her diagnosis. To God alone be the glory!

He Took One Look

For he will command his angels concerning you
to guard you in all your ways. (Psalm 91:11 NIV)

I ENTERED THE patient's room on 2East. At first
glance, all I could see was a head of long, fiery red hair
on an elderly lady. I would quickly come to know her as
Marta. She was busy unpacking and getting things settled
in her room before beginning her treatment for metastatic melanoma. She had come from the Midwest with
her husband Harry, to whom she had been married for
approximately forty years. However, as soon as I heard
her speak, I instantly knew she was not born in America,
much less the Midwest. As I spent the following days,
weeks, and months assigned to her care, I felt privileged
to learn about her life and her love story with Harry.

Marta was born and raised in Austria during the Nazi
invasion of WWII. She shared with me many details
about life growing up with her seven sisters. She told me
how Hitler sent baskets of chocolates and flowers to her
mother for Christmas. He planned to make her and her
sisters into a baby factory during the war to carry out his

evil regime of creating an Aryan race. I had never heard of these horrific plans and found myself speechless as I listened to her tell this story.

In 2019, with all the celebrations and special TV reports on World War II, I saw with my own eyes exactly what Marta had been sharing with me. I watched video footage of places in Germany where they were housing hundreds of newborn babies just as she had described. Thankfully, with the help of the Allied forces, this would never become her nor her sisters' reality.

However, a young American GI was stationed in Austria, and as he told me, "I took one look at her and just knew I was going to marry her."

Indeed, it happened just as he said. Marta left Germany after the war ended and came to America. She became the wife of this soldier who helped rescue her and the world from an evil empire. Harry seemed to be as in love with her now as the day he first laid eyes on her. He was always sitting quietly by her side. I don't recall that he ever missed an opportunity to be with her while she was going through her treatments.

They certainly defined the phrase "opposites attract" because he was very reserved and was a man of few words, but he exemplified a tangible, quiet strength.

On the other hand, she was an extreme extrovert in her mid-sixties, was working full time, and had so much life and vitality she could spin circles around both of us. But most importantly, Marta and Harry loved each other and demonstrated it in their unique way, despite their many differences. Their love was unconditional and inspiring for me to see in action. Instead of trying to change one another, they seemed to have found the grace to rejoice in their differences. She was a pure delight to be with, and there was never a dull moment in her presence. Conversations with her were joyful and always encouraging. She invariably had something interesting to talk about or discuss.

Sadly, after some months of therapy, I found out Marta's disease had progressed, making her no longer eligible for treatments on this trial. I was heartbroken. We both had opened up our lives to each other in a vulnerable situation, knowing that her chances of survival were small. But this is often how life comes to us in the medical profession. We have the opportunity to touch the lives of many people in desperate situations, but only for a short time.

I am reminded of a verse in a song by Lee Ann Womack: "Promise me that you'll give faith a fighting chance, and when you get the choice to sit it out or dance, I hope you dance!" Letting my guard down and letting Marta into my heart gave me the chance to dance. I am so thankful I embraced the opportunity to dance with her in life, even for just a few short moments.

We stayed in touch until the end. After Marta died, Harry told me that right before she breathed her last breath, she said, "Harry, look, look at the angels. They are so beautiful." I held back the tears as I listened and never doubted his words because I knew Marta had a confident faith in her Lord Jesus Christ. She often spoke about God and her belief in him, not her fears, worries, or concerns. It was a gift to spend time with her, and I thank God for those special moments that I will always cherish. Her last moments of life remind me of this beautiful verse: "Precious in the sight of the Lord is the death of his faithful servants" (Psalm 116:15 NIV).

Don't Ever Forget:
God Is Good!

But he said to me, "My grace is sufficient for
you, for my power is made perfect in weakness."
Therefore I will boast all the more gladly of my
weaknesses, so that the power of Christ may rest
upon me. (2 Corinthians 12:9 ESV)

PETER, A DELIGHTFUL twenty-eight-year-old with
a freckled face and red hair, was a husband and the father
of two small children, experiencing the battle of his life
as he suffered from metastatic melanoma. He met his
wife while serving in Christian ministry in the inner city
of Philadelphia. Peter was a fun-loving person with a
playful disposition. I can imagine him being the life of
the party whenever he entered the room.

The treatment of Interleukin therapy (IL2) that he
would receive worked quickly on patients' immune
systems, and the side effects often made them very sick.
Almost immediately with the first infusion, patients
could experience nausea, vomiting, diarrhea, shaking
chills, water retention, and skin irritation to some

degree. I mention all this because I distinctly remember Peter cracking a joke in the middle of being sick on his stomach. I've never met anyone who could do that. But this was his personality, his way of coping with a horrible situation.

He also had a deep abiding faith in Jesus Christ. One day after his wife and two children had been visiting with him, he said to me, "I told my son, no matter what happens to me, don't ever forget that God is good!" I could tell by his sincerity and the strength in his voice that he meant it with all his heart.

It was beautiful for me to hear him say these words, and it was also convicting at the same time. Peter was facing death head-on, praying for healing, suffering through medical treatments, yet proclaiming through it all, "God is good!" This is Christianity at its core. Jesus said, "I have told you these things, so that in me you may have peace. In this world you will have trouble. But take heart! I have overcome this world" (John 16:33 NIV). He never promised he would deliver us from all suffering, but that he would never leave us alone in our trials.

One morning, I was in Peter's room giving him some medication in his IV to help treat his symptoms before hanging his next dose of Interleukin 2. As he was lying in bed, half awake and half asleep, he acknowledged me but mostly lay there without stirring. I returned to his room a little later that morning when he was fully awake to see how he was doing. He proceeded to tell me, "When you were in here earlier, I wasn't sure if I was dreaming or awake, but I saw this lady with light gray hair wearing a white lab coat intently watching everything you were doing. She had a nametag on her coat and the letters spelled the word 'FAITH.'"

I was pretty busy that morning as usual, so I quietly listened and said, "Wow, she must have been your guardian angel," not thinking much about it.

He smiled back and said, "Yeah, maybe so."

That evening as I drove home after my shift, I always had time to reflect on the day because of the slow-moving traffic along the 495 corridor between Bethesda, Maryland, and Northern Virginia. As I rehearsed the day's events and what Peter had said, I concluded that FAITH was probably my guardian angel. And only heaven knows how much I needed her help in my day to day work as a nurse.

The following morning when I entered Peter's room, the first thing out of his mouth was, "I think Faith was your guardian angel."

We looked each other in the eyes and smiled, and I answered, "You know, I think you are right!"

God had given Peter grace to face an impossible situation. He had also sent an angel to help me do what seemed, at times, to be an impossible job. The emotional and physical toll on us as oncology nurses was tremendous. We went from room to room each day, giving all we had to try and help our patients heal and get well. We became their home away from home. We loved them, and they loved us. When one of our patients died, we all grieved. But many of us clung to the truth that hope is not just for this life. Heaven is real and waiting for everyone who chooses to trust in Jesus, as Peter did.

I'll Show You Jerusalem

I saw the Holy City, the new Jerusalem, coming
down out of heaven from God, prepared as a bride
beautifully dressed for her husband. (Revelation
21:2 NIV)

JOSH, A YOUNG Israeli man from Jerusalem in his
early twenties, came to our hospital accompanied by his
father to seek experimental therapy for his brain tumor.
I don't recall if the cancer originated in his brain tissue
or if the primary tumor started somewhere else and
spread to his brain. But I remember that his disease was
very aggressive because he stayed with us only a week or
two and then was discharged to return to Israel with no
further options in our care.

Looking back, I can see how miraculous it was that
we could connect so quickly. There is typically not much
small talk when someone is facing a terminal illness. It
is easy to take care of the patient's physical needs, but
allowing oneself to invest emotionally is a different
story. Life at every age is precious, but caring for young
people with cancer is even more challenging because it is

bewildering to grasp that they will die without having the opportunity to live out their lives.

Several days before he would leave our hospital, Josh mentioned that he was very anxious about getting on such a long flight to Israel. He had been experiencing severe headaches and was concerned about the change in cabin pressure and its consequences on him during his flight. It must have been the Lord who gave me this idea—I decided to call EL Al, the Israeli Airline, and explain the situation about his fears. I was so thrilled when they told me they would help him out and elated when I eventually discovered they had upgraded him and his father to first class for the entire flight home. This was a time before HIPAA regulations, so it wasn't a problem to mention his name, explain the situation, and ask for a favor—a simple act of kindness to help out a dying person. Sadly, because we now have such strict rules about patient confidentiality, it would take an act of Congress to help a patient like this in today's world. However, at the time, I was so thankful for what they did, and so was he.

Before Josh left, we had several opportunities to talk about life, faith, and death. He shared with me that he had been exploring the beliefs of other religions besides his Jewish faith. We discussed foundational truths about Christianity, and with his permission, I shared my faith in Jesus Christ. I had been given a book by another patient entitled *A Man Named Jesus* and asked Josh if he would be interested in taking it to Jerusalem to read. He gladly accepted my offer.

Several weeks later, some of my colleagues working the evening shift told me I had missed a phone call from Josh's cousin living in Tel Aviv. He wanted to thank me for helping him get a comfortable flight home. I hated missing this call but was so excited to hear it was an uneventful trip for him and his dad. Getting an international phone call at work was a big deal in the era when we didn't have cell phones.

Not long after this call, I received a letter from Josh. Thankfully, after all these years, I saved his letter and will never forget one of the sentences he wrote: "Maybe someday, I will show you the New Jerusalem." My heart skipped a beat when I read his words. I believe this was a prophetic statement. And I also pray it will happen just as he described in his letter. God indeed promises to make ALL things new one day!

Don't Be Afraid to Call

And if I go and prepare a place for you, I will come back and take you to be with me that you also may be where I am. (John 14:3 NIV)

CHRIS WAS A handsome man in his mid- to late thirties, interesting to converse with, fun to be around, and fighting to beat his metastatic melanoma. He was Canadian, but he used to work as a chef in Santa Monica, California. There he met his wife Cindy, who was waiting tables at the same restaurant. She shared with me that when she and Chris met, they were both in unhappy relationships. They decided to end those, and the two of them started dating. Several years later, they were married, moved back to Canada, and had several children. Cindy was homeschooling them, so they were always able to be at the hospital for weeks at a time while Chris received his IL2 treatments.

They were an adorable couple and perfectly fitted for each other. Both of them readily talked about their Christian faith. Even though Cindy exhibited tremendous strength, I could tell she was quietly suffering as she sat by the side of her friend and husband. She stoically watched him endure the difficult side effects of the immunotherapy, which was at the same time giving them hope for a cure. In marriage, the Bible says, "Two shall become one flesh," and I witnessed this over and over with couples when spouses came to sit night and day at the bedside of their loved ones. Once when talking with Cindy, she mentioned to me that Chris loved photography and watching Sunday afternoon football games. But when he was diagnosed with metastatic cancer, he turned off the TV and began pouring himself into finishing his photography projects in order to leave something of himself behind for his family.

After patients would finish a cycle of immunotherapy treatments, they would return home to completely recover. They would then be scheduled for CT scans about four to six weeks later and would meet with the doctors in the clinic to determine if the cancerous tumors were responding to therapy or growing larger. If the therapy was working, they would be scheduled to begin a new round of treatments. If there was no regression of the cancer, then sadly, they would be discharged from the trial.

Sometimes our patients who did not have a response would come by to visit the nursing staff on 2East to thank us personally for our care and to say goodbye. Some of them would give us their phone numbers and invite us to stay in touch, as Cindy and Chris did with me. It was emotionally painful to watch our patients, who often came to feel like dear friends, suffer through these treatments. It was even more painful to find out their tumors were growing and they would not be returning for more therapy. We always knew that we were their last hope for a cure because they had already completed standard therapies that were FDA approved for their type of cancer before coming to the NIH. Essentially, we all knew in our hearts that we were saying farewell to someone who most likely was going home to die.

So I said goodbye to Chris and Cindy with hugs, holding back tears with the promise to stay in touch. Over the next several months, I did indeed call to say hello and see how Chris was doing. The last time I remember calling, I waited longer than before because I could not face the inevitability that one day when I called, he would not be on the other end of the phone.

When Chris did answer, he did not beat around the bush; nor was he afraid to speak of his death. He boldly said to me, "It's hard for you to call, isn't it, Tammy?"

I answered him, "I am sorry. Yes, it is hard."

Then he said to me with confident faith and assurance, "So when you call again and I am not here, you know where I will be, and one day we will see each other again."

He was facing death head-on, and yet it was his unwavering faith that was giving comfort to me that day. I know that Chris is in heaven today, and I know where I am going when I die.

What about you? Jesus promises everyone that if you believe in him, he goes and prepares a place for us and we will be with him forever. No one is too far away from the Lord that his arm cannot reach. But don't wait for him to come to you. He already did that on a Roman cross 2,000 years ago. The book of James, written by the brother of Jesus, tells us to "Come near to God and he will come near to you" (James 4:8 NIV).

The Little Things

For the sake of Jacob My servant, and Israel My
chosen one. (Isaiah 45:4 NASB)

THE START OF a new shift came fast and furious at 6
A.M. on 2East. There were new patients to meet, new chal-
lenges to face, and new experiences to be encountered
with people just outside our conference room where we
would get reports before starting the day. I walked into
the sterile hospital room with no pretty decorations or
designer fabrics, and I saw a beautiful Israeli woman with
long, flowing locks of curly blonde hair and her equally
beautiful twenty-year-old daughter lying on the bed.

Sasha had a very rare form of sarcoma, a type of
cancer that has its beginning in the cells of our soft
tissue. It can develop in many different locations in the
body. There are fewer than 200,000 cases each year in
the United States. Sasha and her mom had come from
Jerusalem to seek experimental treatment at the National
Cancer Institute. Here was a mother and her daughter
far from home, alone in a big medical center, and facing
a health crisis while clinging to hope.

Years ago, the world wasn't as small as it is today, and meeting people from other countries felt exotic. It was fascinating to learn about other lifestyles and cultures from around the world. Probably because of my love of travel, I easily bonded with them both, and it helped that they were super friendly. After several days of taking care of Sasha and interacting with her mom, who never left her side, I realized that the American diet was quite different from what they were used to in Israel. So one day I asked them, "What would a typical Israeli breakfast consist of?" I sincerely had no idea. I listened carefully, taking note of exactly what they told me. The next day I was able to surprise them with a very finely chopped cucumber, tomato, and onion salad, hard-boiled eggs, bread, and cheese. I could never have imagined how such a small gesture could bring so much delight until I saw their faces.

I had brought them a tiny piece of their culture to this foreign country they were visiting, and it clearly made them feel welcomed in America. As we all know, food often has that effect on each of us when we travel throughout the world. We will look for familiar meals that make us feel at home. For that exact reason, many Americans like to eat at McDonald's when traveling abroad. For me, it was a simple task—I didn't even have to cook, and yet they seemed so happy. It is astounding that sometimes the simplest acts of kindness can have a profound effect on us as human beings. It does seem to be true that the little things we do for others can make the biggest difference.

Sasha was very physically fit and had served in the Israeli Defense Forces before she got sick. Israel is one of only a few countries in the world that has a mandatory military service requirement for women. Female combat soldiers are required to serve two years and four months and continue in the reserves up to age thirty-eight. I will never forget seeing a female soldier while traveling in Jerusalem in 1997. We were attending a public event when I looked up and saw a young woman standing guard with other soldiers near our area. But it was most striking to see her long, dark ponytail and something like an AK-47 strapped to her back. Some images are forever planted in our memories, and this is one of them for me.

I had a lot of respect for what Sasha had been through and how she had served her country. She had a strong spirit and exhibited a deep determination to get well and beat her cancer. Unfortunately, she did not get better and had to return to Israel. Upon leaving, her mom gave me their contact information and insisted that I get in touch with them if ever I had the chance to visit their country.

Of course, at the time I never imagined I would be visiting Israel, but fast forward several years, and I was enrolled in a course at Georgetown University called the Arab Israeli Conflict. My professor, Ehud Sprinzak, a world-renowned expert on terrorism, was from the Hebrew University of Jerusalem and had served in the Six-Day War in 1967. It was thrilling to sit under the teaching of a man who had personally lived and experienced biblical prophecy come true. I had so much admiration for him as a professor, an Israeli soldier, a political scholar, and an author.

Part of the requirement to complete the course was to write a paper as a final project in the class, and he suggested that I write one on the Balfour Declaration. This Declaration was part of the process of how Israel would become a nation in 1947, which God had said would happen when he called Abraham to leave his country in Ur of the Chaldeans and settle in the land of Canaan several thousands of years earlier. You are probably wondering how all these dots connect, but hang with me.

Taking care of Sasha, meeting her mom, and enrolling in this course sparked my interest in visiting Israel. Plus, the foundations of my Christian faith all started in this region of the Middle East. Within a four-week time-frame, I had signed up with a Christian tour company and was headed to Israel. It was all very exciting until I was standing in line at JFK Airport trying to board my El Al flight to the Holy Land. They have multiple levels of security, and rightly so, but it's not what we were used to in the 1990s. I was questioned for two and a half hours by multiple people in El Al security because I had borrowed a friend's luggage, knew someone in Jerusalem, and had planned this trip within one month. These combined events put up red flags in their minds. After being strip searched respectfully and having my luggage unpacked piece by piece, I was put back together and personally escorted to my seat on the plane. By this time, I was in tears even though I knew I had done nothing wrong and was certainly not a terrorist.

In the end, it was a small price to pay for an abso-lutely wonderful experience in the Holy Land. Visiting sites such as the birthplace of Jesus and the Garden of Gethsemane, placing prayers in the Wailing Wall, floating in the Dead Sea, and visiting many other places—all of these experiences were more than I could have imagined.

I was also able to meet and spend a few moments with Sasha's mother at the Children's Holocaust Memorial where she worked. She was happy to see me, but since we had been together last, Sasha had died, and it was a bittersweet meeting. I couldn't imagine how she could work in such a sad place, but somehow I wondered if maybe she felt a connection to all the mothers who had lost their children. I once heard NCI Chief Dr. Stephen Rosenberg say, "Cancer is like the Holocaust; it takes the lives of so many innocent victims."

She Played the Piano

Weeping may endure for a night, but joy comes
in the morning. (Psalm 30:5 NKJV)

CAROLINE WAS A very attractive woman with fair
skin and blonde hair. She was a morning TV host in one
of the southern states. We have all heard the expression
"Sweet Georgia Peach," and Caroline personified this
with everything in her being. Nothing but pure kindness
exuded from her every pore and word she spoke, and
her kindness quickly touched everyone who was lucky
enough to be in her presence. She looked elegant and
acted with such poise that at some point in her life she
may have been a beauty contestant. I don't know this for
a fact, but she definitely had all the qualities of one.

When I met Caroline, she had already been a patient
on 2East, and all the nurses who took care of her before
me adored this southern beauty. She had been through
IL2 treatments and had experienced success in the
regression of her melanoma. But now she was back in
Bethesda, and the melanoma had reared its ugly head
in a lymph node under her left arm. There was a lot of

discussion among the surgeons concerning the best way to treat this new occurrence. The team would meet for a conference every Friday morning to explore all options for each patient being presented. Should they remove it surgically or give her more IL2 in hopes of shrinking the tumor and eradicate any other spread of cancer cells that might be lurking in places that did not show up on CT scans?

They decided surgery would be the best option to remove it and hopefully give Caroline a better chance of survival. Sadly, with cancer, there are no 100 percent guarantees. These physicians and research scientists dedicated their lives to treating and finding new and novel modalities to help cure people with cancer. These decisions about each patient came from years of experience and some of the brightest minds in the field. Dr. Stephen Rosenberg, chief of the NCI Surgery Branch, is a pioneer in immunotherapy treatments for cancer. This was the caliber of professionalism on her team. He and everyone else making these decisions visited their patients every morning, knew them personally, and cared deeply about them.

The team made the recommendation for surgery, and Caroline agreed to have it done. For a while, it seemed to be a good choice, and things were going well. But over time, the tumor started growing back in the same left arm. And for some unknown reason, it became worse than ever. She came back for more IL2, but nothing was stopping the spread. Her arm became so swollen she no longer had use of it. Once again, I was almost crippled with sadness because she was a young single woman like me, and we had become close acquaintances. She was originally from my home state and would often stay with her mother in between her trips to Maryland.

After she was discharged from our hospital, she moved in with her mother, and we would talk from time to time on the phone. Caroline's sincere faith in Christ gave her the confidence that she would be in heaven when she died. At the same time, she never gave up on living and believing in God's power to heal. Eventually, she did "fall asleep," as Scripture tells us, a young woman in the prime of her life and stunningly gorgeous. One would think that cancer had the last word in her life, but it did not.

Several months after her death, I called her mother, and as we chatted, I soon realized where Caroline got her southern charm. Her mom was just as gracious and kind as Caroline. We talked about all that had happened, and as I expressed my sincerest condolences, her mom proceeded to tell me about a dream she had. She shared with me that Caroline used to play the piano. In her dream, she saw her seated and playing. At one particular moment in the dream, Caroline turned toward her mother sideways on the piano bench with a huge, beautiful smile on her face and played the piano with only her left hand, as if to say, "Don't worry, Mom, I am alive. I am living and happy, no longer suffering, and doing what I love to do." Just as God allowed Marta to see angels before she died, I am convinced that he also gave Caroline's mother this dream to comfort and help her grieve the loss of her daughter.

Jesus promises us all eternal life if we believe in him and in his promises. "Let not your heart be troubled; believe in God, believe also in me. In my Father's house are many rooms: if it were not so, would I have told you that I go to prepare a place for you? And when I go and prepare a place for you, I will come again and take you to myself, that where I am you may be also" (John 14:1–3 RSV).

The Jewish Rabbi

The Lord is close to the broken hearted and saves
those who are crushed in spirit. (Psalm 34:18 NIV)

ISAAC HAD ESCAPED Nazi Germany as a young child
during WWII. Some years later, he managed to travel to
New York City, where he eventually found work and met
his wife, who had also fled from the war. Isaac lived in
NYC for many years, working and enjoying his life.

As he lay in his hospital bed suffering from metastatic renal cell cancer, he shared with me how his entire
family had died during the Holocaust. He didn't go into
any details, but his one sentence with few words revealed
a lifetime of pain and sorrow. Isaac was a gentleman,
very kind with a pleasant demeanor, and he went out
of his way to make sure he never bothered anyone. He
never drew attention to himself, seemingly accepting
whatever came his way without complaining and with a
calm strength, except when his wife was around. He tried
to hide his feelings from her because he told me, "She
gets so anxious and worried, and then she makes me so
nervous." I knew he meant well and that he truly loved

her. I think he didn't have the strength to comfort her emotionally while getting his treatments. Considering all they had been through together, I sensed that it was difficult for him to see her in such distress.

One Sunday evening, as I was taking care of him, I noticed he was particularly talkative and joyful while awaiting a visit from his rabbi, who was driving down from NYC. I remember thinking what a special individual he must be to his Jewish congregation for this rabbi to drive four or five hours for a visit, turn around, and drive back the same night. It was intriguing for me also because I had just watched a movie called *A Stranger Among Us* where Melanie Griffin plays an undercover cop. In the film, she lives with an Orthodox Jewish community in New York to try and solve a murder mystery in the Diamond District. I was so fascinated by the cultural aspects of Orthodox Jewish people based on this movie that I couldn't wait to get a few minutes to interact with his rabbi to understand how much of the film was actually true or just a Hollywood version.

After he visited Isaac, I did indeed get the opportunity to meet the rabbi. He was much younger than I had expected and very eager to engage in conversation. I found out that many things portrayed in the movie about Hasidic Jews were true. At the time, I was curious about some of the teachings of Kabbalah. They believe that when God made souls and sends them to earth, they split apart upon entering this world. And if you meet the person you are destined to be with in life, then you have found your "soul mate."

I am in no position to verify or debate this teaching, but at the time, it seemed to be a beautiful idea, especially since I was hoping to find romance in my own life. My conversation with the rabbi was a delightful exchange of our personal views and understandings of biblical and modern-day Jewish culture and beliefs, along with an injection of my protestant faith. No pun intended. This interaction could only have happened late into an evening shift because the day shifts were super busy with new admissions, discharges, and care of sometimes very sick patients. As you can see, our hospital was like a microcosm of the United Nations, with patients, nurses, scientists, and physicians from all over America and different parts of the world.

Once I was taking care of a charming gentleman from Ukraine when a surgical resident walking by casually mentioned, "Your patient is possibly one of the smartest mathematicians in the world."

Curiously, I asked him, "How do you know?"

He proceeded to tell me, "Because I was studying to be a math major before I went into medicine."

Every patient I encountered was an opportunity to step into the universe of another soul, marvel at the creative genius of our maker God, and learn about their life stories while enhancing my own simply by taking the time to stop and listen. Nothing has changed. Listening and being genuinely interested in other people's lives is a gift of kindness we can offer to those we encounter.

I once heard that when people would meet with the world-renowned evangelist, the late Reverend Billy Graham, he rarely talked about his own life. Instead, he wanted to hear only about theirs. The brother of Jesus wrote, "My dear brothers and sisters, take note of this: Everyone should be quick to listen, slow to speak and slow to become angry" (James 1:19 NIV). Oh, how life would be so much sweeter if we all—me included—could put these words into practice more often. It's never too late to start!

I continued to be Isaac's nurse, but I don't recall him being on our unit for very long. It's strange how some people, even though our encounters are brief, can leave lasting impressions on our lives and in our hearts. He was one of those people, and I am ever so thankful to have met Mr. Isaac.

A Twinkle in Her Eye

The LORD directs the steps of the godly. He delights in every detail of their lives. (Psalm 37:23 NLT)

SUE WAS A very thoughtful, unobtrusive, middle-aged lady from a small city in Virginia, and she was in the hospital with metastatic renal cell carcinoma. Compared to many of my patients, our time together was brief, but she tremendously impacted my life. If I remember correctly, she was divorced and usually came alone for her treatments, or she had a few friends popping in and out for short periods. Even though she was very reserved and quite introverted, she had a quick-witted sense of humor that I had the opportunity to witness whenever we had the chance to engage in conversation.

I always tried to find some common ground to connect with my patients, helping to put them at ease and making our time together more enjoyable for both of us. How horrible to be sick and not particularly like the person taking care of you, which would add extra stress that no one needs.

I had just been reading a fascinating book called *A Severe Mercy*, a real-life love story full of wonder and hope by Sheldon Vanauken, a professor at Lynchburg College. Because I found out that Sue was from a city close to Lynchburg, I proceeded to discuss this book with her, going on and on about how it was the most intriguingly romantic book I had ever read. I was totally enamored with this author, and at one point in his career, he studied at the University of Oxford, England, and became personal friends with C.S. Lewis. Lewis was the very famous British writer, professor of English literature at Oxford, lay theologian, and best known for his works of fiction, such as *The Screwtape Letters* and *The Chronicles of Narnia*, and his nonfiction Christian apologetics, such as *Mere Christianity*.

As I continued to discuss my love for this book and author, I could see this little twinkle in Sue's eyes and a sly grin come across her face. I remember catching myself mid-sentence and asking, "Why do you have such a funny grin on your face?" She couldn't hold back her excitement any longer when she blurted out that she personally knew Sheldon Vanauken and had worked with him for years. I was absolutely speechless. How often do you get to meet someone who works with and personally knows the author of your current favorite book?

Now the walls came down, and I bonded instantly with her by an author, a book, and a college in Lynchburg, Virginia. This seemed to be so much more than just a patient-nurse relationship. It felt like a divine appointment from heaven. As a Christian, I don't believe in chance happenings or coincidences. I believe God orders our steps and connects the dots to the circumstances of our lives. He alone does the supernatural work, but we get to experience such pleasure when we are consciously aware of what he is doing. In the words of C.S. Lewis, we find ourselves "surprised by joy."

Sue was a lovely person, and I thoroughly enjoyed being her nurse. Sadly, she was not a patient of ours for very long because the treatment did not work as we had hoped, and our time together was short-lived. We kept in touch through writing letters. Unexpectedly, one day while at work, I received a package from her right around the time of my birthday. I excitedly opened the box, and inside was a signed copy of Shelden Vanauken's book, *A Severe Mercy*, addressed to me personally. It was one of the best birthday gifts I have ever received.

I felt so privileged and honored by Sue's kind gesture when she was going through such a significant health crisis. Through the years, I have realized that simply taking a few extra minutes in getting to know someone can open up a rich treasure of shared interests and common bonds. And at the end of the day, I think we can all agree that life's most precious moments are the ones shared with others.

Sue was a quiet, gentle, and generous soul. This passage comes to mind when I think of her: "Your beauty should not come from outward adornment, such as elaborate hairstyles and the wearing of gold jewelry or fine clothes. Rather, it should be that of your inner self, the unfading beauty of a gentle and quiet spirit, which is of great worth in God's sight" (1 Peter 3:3–4 NIV).

All Alone One Night

Everyone who calls on the name of the Lord will
be saved. (Romans 10:13 NIV)

MR. STOCKFORD WAS a unique character in many
ways, and sadly one that several of the nurses found hard
to get along with and challenging to care for. He was an
elderly gentleman with a slender, tall physique, and he
was often disgruntled. He suffered from a late stage of
cancer called mesothelioma that affected his lungs. He
certainly never wanted to find himself at the NIH under-
going experimental therapy at the end of his life. After
having surgery to remove a large portion of the tumor,
he agreed to a Phase 1 Clinical Trial that required him to
stay many days and weeks on our unit.

He always came alone and was estranged from his
children and divorced from their mother. Most of the
time, he had an irritable demeanor and never seemed
to care if people knew exactly how he felt. He reminded
me of Ebenezer Scrooge. Please don't think I am rude in
the way I describe him—hang with me because this story

and his personality get better, but it took some time and patience on both of our parts.

Unexpectedly, I found myself being Mr. Stockford's primary care nurse, meaning that he would be permanently assigned to me when I was on duty. This type of nursing practice ensured continuity of care with our patients. I believe in providential guidance, but I can honestly say I don't always recognize it when it comes my way. I didn't particularly want to spend so much time with this sometimes grumpy and rude elderly patient. However, without a doubt, God had put us together, and I even found myself, over time, beginning to honestly like him.

As I prayed for him, I began to see past his superficial hard covering. I recognized a lonely, sad, and isolated dying person trying to cope and navigate a crisis all alone. Isn't this often the case when we begin to pray for the seemingly unpleasant people in our lives? I have found that the Lord usually changes me first, and then, sometimes they follow. After weeks of spending ten-hour days in and out of his room, the barriers began to break down, and he slowly started to trust me.

It makes me chuckle to remember an incident once when he stood in his room and asked in sort of an irritated and puzzled tone, "Tammy, why do you have to be so nice to me?"

I replied honestly, "I don't know. I guess because God wants me to."

This was the work of the Holy Spirit, enabling me to love this seemingly unlovable man. And if we are sincere, this is the kind of love Jesus offers to each of us: his unconditional love.

Days, weeks, and months went by as Mr. Stockford continued with his treatments. He confessed to me one day that he had not been a good husband nor a good father. Admitting that he had lived his life thinking only of himself, he deeply regretted this now. He needed his family, but he was so difficult to deal with that I can understand why they never came around.

I hated doing shiftwork with a passion, because for the first night, I would be awake for twenty-six hours straight, and for me, it felt brutal. If you have ever worked the night shift, you know exactly what I am talking about. I had never been one to stay up late, so around 4 A.M. I would literally feel as if I were going to keel over and collapse. One of our young nurses would pop pieces of chocolate candy in her mouth all night to stay awake. It reminded me of the famous scene from *I Love Lucy* when

Lucy and Ethel were working in the chocolate factory. We all needed something to push through the agony of sleep deprivation.

But this particular night was different. Mr. Stockford was down the hall away from the nurse's station and had a room all to himself, an unusual situation because there were no private rooms on our unit. We must have had a low census that evening.

As I made rounds checking on all my assigned patients, I came to his room around midnight. He was still awake and sitting on the edge of his bed. He started telling me he felt that he had been such a terrible person all his life, and I could sense he was truly remorseful.

What happened next took me totally by surprise. Without thinking, I said to him, "Why don't you confess to the Lord that you are sorry; he will understand."

Suddenly, he began to sob with deep anguish and cried out, "My God, my God, I am so sorry, I am so sorry."

As I stood there, shocked and speechless, completely caught off guard by what I was witnessing, I knew that based on what the Bible tells us, Mr. Stockford's eternal destiny had changed in an instant. God hears the prayers of the sincerely repentant and promises them eternal life if they turn from their sins and receive salvation in Jesus Christ, a gift freely offered to everyone.

I stayed by his side, listening, talking with him, and explaining to him that what he had just prayed changed everything based on what God tells us in the Bible. He could not remove his past mistakes, but his decision to cry out to God changed his future for all eternity.

Unfortunately, Mr. Stockfod was discharged from the hospital because of progressive disease. But I found out through our social worker that he had been reunited with his son. He and his wife had taken him home to be with them before he died. A lifetime of regrets now had a beautiful ending. He received the grace to enjoy a restored relationship with his family and his Redeemer and Savior, Jesus Christ.

God is always reaching out to us! As Jesus hung on the cross for the sins of the world, one of the criminals hanging beside him said, "'Jesus, remember me when you come into your kingdom.' Jesus answered him, 'Truly I tell you, today you will be with me in paradise'" (Luke 23:42–43 NIV).

She Never Stopped Laughing

Do not grieve, for the joy of the LORD is your
strength. (Nehemiah 8:10 NIV)

BETSY WAS THE epitome of a southern belle. She had
an infectious accent that kept us hanging on every word
she said. It was melodious, like an Italian dialect. She was
the friendly neighbor we wanted to sit with on the front
porch during a hot Sunday afternoon, drinking sweet tea
and chatting until the sun slid down beyond the horizon.
Betsy was funny and a little mischievous. She had a
twinkle in her eye, and that contagious laughter of hers
would fill up the room.

Her deep faith made her face light up every time she
spoke about Jesus. She loved the Lord and was never
ashamed or shy about sharing with a nurse, doctor, or
another patient about her Savior and friend, Jesus Christ.
She was someone who prayed without ceasing and never
stopped believing that God would heal her. I think he
did heal her of metastatic melanoma after many treatments of Interleukin 2 therapy and multiple surgeries.
However, it seemed as if God kept her coming back to

the NIH because she was such a powerful witness to everyone about her faith.

Once, she was asked to appear in a large conference room filled with many prestigious surgeons discussing and planning her next treatment options. As she sat quietly on stage by herself in front of the audience, at one point she humbly and innocently proclaimed that she was praying for them. To face a room full of highly educated people and declare her faith in God took courage. She did it boldly, just as Saint Paul wrote: "But God chose the foolish things of this world to shame the wise: God chose the weak things of the world to shame the strong" (1 Corinthians 1:27 NIV).

Betsy was very close to her family, and on many occasions, her sister Julie would drive with her from Tennessee to spend several weeks by her side while she underwent treatments. Even though they were sisters, they acted like two little schoolgirls, always laughing, giggling, and looking for opportunities to see the fun in life amidst the deep suffering and sorrow they were experiencing. Theirs was indeed a special relationship, and, thankfully, they felt like the sisters I never had.

I guess being from the South, sharing the same faith, and laughing about the things we had in common just molded our hearts together. We all knew that the only way to drink sweet tea was with tons of sugar and freshly squeezed lemon juice. And, of course, the best ice cream was homemade on a hot summer afternoon shared with family and friends as we took our turn churning the old-fashioned hand crank ice cream maker, which in my opinion, made it taste so much better. If you don't know what this is, look it up on Amazon. Everybody needs one of these.

By taking care of Betsy for so many days, I also got to know her tenderhearted father, son, daughter-in-law, and grandchildren. There were endless conversations about each one of them. Sometimes, however, she had to come for her treatments by herself. By then, I had taken a new position as a research nurse and had regular working hours. I would frequently stop by her room on my way home to sit and chat for a minute. She trusted me as her nurse and now as her friend and would often open up about the complexities of family relationships. These situations in life are common to all of us. However, at the end of the day, family meant everything to her. If they could not be close physically, they were near to her heart because she never stopped talking about them. It was such a pleasure to sit by her side and mostly listen, because despite all she was going through, and it was a lot, she never complained and never once missed an opportunity to pray for me or anyone else who had a need. Betsy was filled with the Holy Spirit from head to toe and lived her life following his lead as best she could.

After coming to the NIH for several years of experimental therapies, she was discharged from our care. She no longer had evidence of melanoma in her body. However, through letters and phone calls, I found out she was diagnosed with another type of cancer some years later and eventually died from this disease.

Even though my heart was aching for her loss, I knew her body was laid to rest in this life while her soul was more alive than ever. "Precious in the sight of the LORD is the death of his faithful servants" (Psalm 116:15 NIV).

I am confident that one day Betsy, Julie, and I will meet again in the presence of our Lord and Savior, Jesus Christ, to worship and adore him, and to laugh again with no more heartaches, suffering, or tears. This is what the Bible promises to all of those who put their faith in Christ.

May I ask, who and what have you put your faith in? Do you know where you will spend eternity? God doesn't force himself on anyone but gives each of us a choice.

In which direction are your daily choices and decisions leading you?

"This day I call the heavens and the earth as witnesses against you that I have set before you life and death, blessings and curses. Now choose life, so that you and your children may live and that you may love the LORD your God, listen to his voice, and hold fast to him. For the Lord is your life, and he will give you many years in the land he swore to give to your fathers, Abraham, Isaac and Jacob" (Deuteronomy 30:19–20 NIV).

My Mom Is in Heaven

"For I know the plans I have for you," declares the LORD, "plans to prosper to you and not to harm you, plans to give you hope and a future." (Jeremiah 29:11 NIV)

AS I ENTERED the narthex of St. Alban's Chapel next to the Washington National Cathedral in Washington, D.C., I was greeted by the smiling face of Catherine's middle son. He seemed genuinely happy that I had come to attend his mother's funeral service. It was hard for me to imagine that he could manage to exhibit joy in these sad circumstances at such a young age. However, as we exchanged greetings and I expressed my condolences, he quickly responded with complete confidence that he knew his mom was in heaven, and one day he would see her again.

I had come to know Catherine, in the same way I got to know many of my other patients—by a phone conversation with her physician who was trying to get her enrolled in our study. She was a lovely woman, a foreign language teacher at a local private school in the

D.C. area, who, along with teaching, led her students on study abroad programs in Europe.

After speaking several times on the phone and getting all the necessary study results, I set her up for a clinic visit. I don't know about you, but after talking to people on the phone, I usually try to imagine how they will look by the sound of their voice. When I meet them in person, they rarely match what I had conjured up in my mind, but Catherine indeed looked like the person I had imagined. She was delightful, gracious, soft-spoken, and petite.

Despite having a large tumor in her liver, she met the study protocol and was set up for our liver perfusion surgery. We never gave the patients hope for a total cure, but we wanted everyone who came on the study to know that there was a very good chance, based on the evidence of other patients' results, that their tumor would most likely shrink, and they would have more time with their loved ones. And for Catherine, that meant her husband and three sons.

She was accepted and came through the surgery without any complications. We always brought our patients back to our follow-up clinic to have scans around six weeks after being discharged from the hospital. After reviewing them with the principal investigator, who was also the chief surgeon, it was evident that she did not respond to the therapy, which was very unusual. Both of our hearts sank. I dreaded the moment when we would walk into the room with Catherine and her husband, knowing they were anxiously awaiting answers, hoping and praying with all their hearts it would be good news. I, too, prayed for her as I did for all my patients.

Ray had to deliver the heartbreaking report as I sat and listened. When he told her the therapy did not work, she, unlike most patients, looked him straight in the eye with childlike innocence and asked, "I don't understand; I thought you said there was a good possibility I would have a response. Why didn't this work for me?"

As Ray began to answer her questions, I noticed he was also trying to conceal his sorrowful feelings. It was unusual for a patient to share their intimate emotions and thoughts with us. His response was very comforting as he began to say, "I don't know why it didn't help you. I am truly sorry. I had hoped for and expected a different outcome. We have seen almost all of our patients have a positive response to this therapy. I really don't under-stand what happened."

At that moment, it felt as if time were standing still, and none of us knew what to do next. The pressure of seeing another patient in the clinic was weighing heavily, but I felt frozen in my chair, unable to move. Catherine and her husband had a bomb dropped on them, and we had a clinic full of other patients waiting to be seen.

This job was never easy, but on this particular day, it felt overwhelmingly difficult. Somehow, if we all remained inside the exam room, life continued to feel hopeful, but once the door was open and they walked outside, the reality of her situation would hit them hard.

Life is full of questions and circumstances that don't seem fair or make sense. It is in these experiences where we can find ourselves standing at a crossroad of our faith. Do we trust God with the complex and painful events, or do we go our own way? The ancient prophet Isaiah had these words of hope to give us: "'For my thoughts are not your thoughts, neither are my ways your ways,' declares the LORD" (Isaiah 55:8 NIV).

The next time I spoke with Catherine, she had kindly invited me into her home for a short visit. It was such a peaceful moment, being surrounded by her loving husband and attentive sons. It was a sweet time and a precious memory of quietly sitting in her presence.

Sometimes this is the best gift we can offer to someone who is grieving or suffering. Catherine eventually died, but I believe with all my heart she is smiling down from heaven, in the presence of the Lord, fully alive and enjoying "joie de vivre" because our ultimate hope as Christians is not in this life!

A White Wedding Gown

God opposes the proud but shows favor to the humble. (1 Peter 5:15 NIV)

TEN THOUSAND LETTERS would be sent out across the nation from a little-known office on the second floor of the National Institutes of Health describing a new study called "Isolated Liver Perfusion." And our phones would begin ringing off the hook. This was the era before cell phones, in case you don't understand that statement.

Since I was a research nurse for three prominent surgeons and principal investigators, in essence, I became one of the channels through which many patients would come to be accepted to our studies. The patients themselves or their doctors would call us inquiring about the study, and in turn, we would request all the appropriate qualifying tests to be performed and the results to be sent to us. This needed to be completed and reviewed before we could bring them to our Friday afternoon clinic to meet in person.

Jane had ocular melanoma that spread to her liver after her initial surgery of removing the primary tumor in her eye. Unfortunately, this is a common occurrence of this disease. She and her husband Dan traveled from the West Coast to our clinic to see if she would be eligible for the study. I don't think I have ever met a couple more dedicated to living out their Christian faith than these two. They were both young, in their mid-forties, attractive people who were full of life. They were playful and joyful while no doubt facing the most challenging trial of their marriage together.

When we met, I strangely felt as if I had known them for years. They were never just focused on their problems and fears but sincerely wanted to get to know me, often asking how they could be praying for me. It was bewildering how they could reach out and show concern for so many others when they were facing a life-threatening illness themselves. Because their attitude was to bless others, I witnessed God's grace sustaining them every step of the way.

One day after Jane had her liver perfusion surgery, I stopped by her hospital room to visit for a little while and just happened to glance down at her bare feet. I noticed someone had painted each of her toenails a different color. Immediately, she started to laugh and explain that her sister, who was visiting, had painted them while she was sleeping. This was the loving, playful family she had been born into, a family who could somehow muster the strength to bring some comedy and humor into their suffering and pain.

The writer of the book of James, who is considered a brother of Jesus, tells us: "Consider it pure joy, my brothers and sisters, whenever you face trials of many kinds because you know that the testing of your faith produces perseverance. Let perseverance finish its work so that you may be mature and complete, not lacking anything" (James 1:2–4 NIV). The Lord never expects us to go through trials alone. That is why he promises to give us the Holy Spirit to help us in all of life's difficulties.

Jesus told the Apostle Paul, "My grace is sufficient for you, for my power is made perfect in weakness" (2 Corinthians 12:9 NIV). As I watched Jane and Dan practice these truths of their Christian faith and applied them to their daily struggles, I witnessed an overflowing abundance of joy expressed in their lives.

Jane recovered fully from her surgery, and she had a positive response to the treatment. However, months later, her cancer started to grow again. I spoke to her once over the phone after she had been discharged from the study. As we casually talked about life and her family, she said to me, "I told Dan that when Nicole [their only daughter], grows up and gets married, make sure she has a gorgeous wedding gown; that's so important for every bride." It was just like her to always be thinking of others.

Sometime later, Dan sent me a note informing me of her death. It was so difficult, but somehow by God's grace, I got the courage to call him. I never knew what I was going to say to someone who had just lost the love of his life, his best friend, and the one he had prayed fervently for God to heal. Plus, I had lost a friend, too, and my heart was also aching.

As we talked, I could sense that his faith had never wavered, nor did he seem to doubt or be angry with God. He told me that the Lord had given him a dream before Jane had died. In the dream, he was standing at the altar of a church dressed to be married. Jane was wearing a beautiful wedding gown as she walked down the aisle toward him. As soon as she stopped and stood beside him, she instantly disappeared.

I remember Dan saying this dream had given him much comfort because he felt that even though she had been taken from him, she left to be with the Lord. He also mentioned that the day she died, she suddenly stood up beside the bed, lay back down, and took her last breath. He commented that this was her style of doing things.

Through all they had experienced, their faith and courage were remarkable and such a blessing and encouragement to me as I watched them live it out day by day, never knowing what they would face next. Together, they exhibited a humble attitude as servants of the Lord everywhere they went and with everyone they encountered.

Conclusion

THE TIMELINE OF our life's story can span many years or be over in a few minutes or days. Ultimately, we have little control over when we will take our last breath on this earth. But while we are living, the world would advise us to figure things out on our own, take charge of our destiny, and leave God out. It's the exact opposite of what Jesus wants for you and me. He loves to guide us with his wisdom and discernment for all of life's questions and problems we face.

Did you ever stop to think about the same God who created Mount Everest, the zebra, and the butterfly is not on a distant planet somewhere far away. He is near to anyone who will call on his name. The Bible says that he knows the number of hairs on your head, and he even knows when a sparrow falls to the ground and dies. I find it fascinating that as we all have faced two years of a world pandemic, unprecedented natural disasters, and social unrest, God is revealing more of himself in creation through the discovery of the James Webb Space Telescope. Astronomers are observing things in the universe never before seen by man in the history of the world. This encourages me to believe all the more that there is hope, and God is an ever-present help in our times of need. May I leave you with the most important words I think you will ever hear: Jesus loves you!

The LORD your God is in your midst; he is a warrior who can deliver. He takes great delight in you; he renews you by his love; he shouts for joy over you. (Zephaniah 3:17 NET)

CPSIA information can be obtained
at www.ICGtesting.com
Printed in the USA
BVHW041253020323
659554BV00004B/716